ADOLESCENT DEVELOPMENT AND THE BIOLOGY OF PUBERTY

SUMMARY OF A WORKSHOP ON NEW RESEARCH

Forum on Adolescence

Michele D. Kipke, *Editor*

Board on Children, Youth, and Families
Commission on Behavioral and Social Sciences and Education

National Research Council
Institute of Medicine

NATIONAL ACADEMY PRESS
Washington, D.C.

FORUM ON ADOLESCENCE

DAVID A. HAMBURG (*Chair*), Carnegie Corporation of New York (President Emeritus)
HUDA AKIL, Mental Health Research Institute, University of Michigan, Ann Arbor
CHERYL ALEXANDER, Center for Adolescent Health, Johns Hopkins University
CLAIRE BRINDIS, Institute for Health Policy Studies, Division of Adolescent Medicine, University of California, San Francisco
GREG DUNCAN, Institute for Policy Research, Northwestern University
JACQUELYNNE ECCLES, School of Education, University of Michigan, Ann Arbor
ABIGAIL ENGLISH, Adolescent Health Care Project, National Center for Youth Law, Chapel Hill, North Carolina
EUGENE GARCIA, School of Education, University of California, Berkeley
HELENE KAPLAN, Skadden, Arps, Slate, Meagher, and Flom, New York
IRIS F. LITT, Division of Adolescent Medicine, Stanford University
JOHN MERROW, The Merrow Report, New York
ANNE C. PETERSEN, W.K. Kellogg Foundation, Battle Creek, Michigan
KAREN PITTMAN, International Youth Foundation, Baltimore
ANNE PUSEY, Jane Goodall Institute's Center, University of Minnesota
MICHAEL RUTTER, Institute of Psychiatry, University of London
STEPHEN A. SMALL, Department of Child and Family Studies, University of Wisconsin, Madison
BEVERLY DANIEL TATUM, Office of the Dean, Mt. Holyoke College
CAMILLE ZUBRINSKY CHARLES, Department of Sociology, University of Pennsylvania

BARUCH FISCHHOFF, *Liaison, Council, Institute of Medicine;* Social and Decision Sciences, Carnegie Mellon University
ELEANOR E. MACCOBY, *Liaison, Commission on Behavioral and Social Sciences and Education;* Department of Psychology, Stanford University (emeritus)

Michele D. Kipke, *Director*
Zodie Makonnen, *Associate Director*
Amy Gawad, *Senior Project Assistant*
Elena Nightingale, *Adviser*

BOARD ON CHILDREN, YOUTH, AND FAMILIES

JACK P. SHONKOFF (*Chair*), Heller Graduate School, Brandeis University
DAVID V.B. BRITT, Children's Television Workshop, New York
LARRY BUMPASS, Center for Demography and Ecology, University of Wisconsin, Madison
SHEILA BURKE, John F. Kennedy School of Government, Harvard University
DAVID CARD, Department of Economics, University of California, Berkeley
KEVIN GRUMBACH, Department of Family and Community Medicine, Primary Care Research Center, University of California, San Francisco
MAXINE HAYES, Department of Community and Family Health, Washington State Department of Health
MARGARET HEAGARTY, Department of Pediatrics, Harlem Hospital Center, Columbia University
ALETHA C. HUSTON, Department of Human Ecology, University of Texas, Austin
RENEE JENKINS, Department of Pediatrics and Child Health, Howard University
SHEILA KAMERMAN, School of Social Work, Columbia University
SANDERS KORENMAN, School of Public Affairs, Baruch College
CINDY LEDERMAN, Circuit Court, Juvenile Justice Center, Dade County, Florida
SARA McLANAHAN, Office of Population Research, Princeton University
VONNIE McLOYD, Center for Human Growth and Development, University of Michigan
PAUL NEWACHECK, Institute of Health Policy Studies and Department of Pediatrics, University of California, San Francisco
DEBORAH STIPEK, Graduate School of Education, University of California, Los Angeles
PAUL WISE, Department of Pediatrics, Boston Medical Center

EVAN CHARNEY, *Liaison, Council, Institute of Medicine;* Department of Pediatrics, University of Massachusetts Medical School
RUTH T. GROSS, *Liaison, Board on Health Promotion and Disease Prevention, Institute of Medicine;* Professor of Pediatrics Emerita, Stanford University
ELEANOR E. MACCOBY, *Liaison, Commission on Behavioral and Social Sciences and Education;* Department of Psychology, Stanford University (emeritus)

MICHELE D. KIPKE, *Director*
DEBORAH A. PHILLIPS, *Director* (through July 1998)
EMILY PERKINS, *Project Assistant for Communications*
DRUSILLA BARNES, *Administrative Associate*
ELENA NIGHTINGALE, *Scholar-in-Residence*

WORKSHOP ON NEW RESEARCH ON THE BIOLOGY OF PUBERTY AND ADOLESCENT DEVELOPMENT

Participants

MELVIN GRUMBACH (*Chair*), University of California, San Francisco
DAVID A. HAMBURG, Carnegie Corporation of New York (President Emeritus)
HUDA AKIL, Mental Health Research Institute, University of Michigan
ADRIAN ANGOLD, Duke University Medical Center
CHERYL ALEXANDER, Center for Adolescent Health, Johns Hopkins University
FRANK BIRO, Children's Hospital Medical Center, Cincinnati
CLAIRE BRINDIS, Institute for Health Policy Studies, University of California, San Francisco
JEANNE BROOKS-GUNN, Teachers College, Columbia University
WILLIAM DAMON, Center on Adolescence, Stanford University
GREG DUNCAN, Northwestern University
JACQUELYNNE ECCLES, School of Education, University of Michigan, Ann Arbor
ANKE EHRHARDT, New York State Psychiatric Institute
GLEN ELLIOTT, University of California, San Francisco
ABIGAIL ENGLISH, National Center for Youth Law, Chapel Hill, North Carolina
BARUCH FISCHHOFF, Carnegie Mellon University
JAY GIEDD, National Institute of Mental Health, National Institutes of Health
RUTH GROSS, Professor Emerita, Stanford University
CHRIS HAYWARD, Center on Adolescence, Stanford University
CHARLES IRWIN, University of California, San Francisco
IRIS F. LITT, Stanford University
ELEANOR MACCOBY, Stanford University
ANN MASTEN, Institute of Child Development, Minneapolis
JOHN MERROW, The Merrow Report, New York
ANNE PETERSEN, W.K. Kellogg Foundation, Battle Creek, Michigan
KAREN PITTMAN, International Youth Foundation, Baltimore, Maryland
ANNE PUSEY, Jane Goodall Institute's Center, University of Minnesota
DAVID ROWE, University of Arizona

STEPHEN SMALL, University of Wisconsin, Madison
STEPHEN SUOMI, National Institute of Child Health and Human
    Development, National Institutes of Health
ELIZABETH SUSMAN, Pennsylvania State University
CAROL WORTHMAN, Emory University

MICHELE D. KIPKE, *Director,* Forum on Adolescence
FAITH MITCHELL, *Director,* Division on Social and Economic Studies
ELENA NIGHTINGALE, *Scholar-In-Residence*

Contents

Preface	xi
New Research on Adolescent Development and the Biology of Puberty	1
Changes in the Study of Adolescent Development	3
Key Findings of Recent Studies	8
Research Challenges	13
Policy Challenges	17
Improving Public Understanding	21
Conclusion	25
References	26
Appendix: Workshop Agenda	29

Preface

On March 23 and 24, 1998, the Forum on Adolescence gathered an interdisciplinary group of researchers and practitioners to review the state of knowledge about adolescent development at a workshop entitled *New Research on the Biology of Puberty and Adolescent Development.* This workshop focused both on puberty—a set of physical changes rooted in biology that can be timed and measured—and on adolescence—a more general and gradual coming of age that occupies much of the second decade of life and is, as one researcher has written, "rooted in society" (Crockett and Petersen, 1993:45). Participants represented diverse fields and brought to the workshop knowledge about an exceptionally wide range of research, including the fields of pediatric and adolescent medicine, public health, neuroendocrinology, behavioral genetics, anthropology, psychiatry, psychology, sociology, animal behavior, law, and others. Using this knowledge, participants were asked to address five key questions:

1. What changes have taken place in the knowledge base of adolescent development?
2. What key findings have emerged from recent studies?
3. What are some of the most pressing research challenges?
4. What are the policy implications of this research?
5. Which messages need to be communicated in order to mobilize the public to support the development, health, and well-being of adolescents?

Drawing on participants' presentations and discussions, this workshop summary addresses each of these questions. Of necessity, it reflects the particular emphases of the workshop discussions, as well as specific statements made by participants during the workshop.

It is important to note that this workshop was an effort intended to take stock of the current knowledge base on adolescent development and highlight key findings from recent research. It was also convened to help inform the future work of a new, cross-cutting initiative of the Institute of Medicine and the National Research Council called the Forum on Adolescence. Given limitations of both time and scope, this workshop could not address a variety of issues that are certainly very important when considering the development, health, and well-being of adolescents. Four particular issues that were only touched on briefly during the workshop are the role of genetics and the interaction between genetic, individual, social, and environmental influences on adolescent development; the role of nutrition and dietary habits; the role of sleep to the healthy development of adolescents; and the role of socioeconomic status, family income, and poverty on adolescent development. The fact that they were not discussed should not suggest that they are not important issues, nor that they are issues undeserving of consideration.

It is also important to note that this workshop report summarizes material presented and discussed at the workshop. Although it references published materials suggested or provided by participants, it is not intended to provide a comprehensive or thorough review of the field. It is our hope that this report will help to illuminate important issues in the field of adolescent development that deserve further attention and consideration.

We offer our appreciation to all of the presenters and participants for their time and contributions. Special thanks go to the planning group—Huda Akil, Jeanne Brooks-Gunn, Anne Petersen, Anne Pusey, and Elizabeth Susman—who gave freely of their time to set the agenda, select participants, contribute to the meeting, and review the initial draft of the report. A special note of appreciation is due Melvin Grumbach, chair of the planning group, for his thoughtful attention and continual assistance in planning and running the workshop. Thanks are also due to Rima Shore for a distillation of the major themes that emerged from the workshop in her work on this summary report, and to Amy Gawad for her assistance in preparing the document prior to publication. Carnegie Corporation of New York provided support for this activity through its core funding of the Forum on Adolescence.

This report has been reviewed in draft form by individuals chosen for their diverse perspectives and technical expertise, in accordance with procedures approved by the NRC's Report Review Committee. The purpose of this independent review is to provide candid and critical comments that will assist the institution in making the published report as sound as possible and to ensure that the report meets institutional standards for objectivity, evidence, and responsiveness to the study charge. The review comments and draft manuscript remain confidential to protect the integrity of the deliberative process.

We wish to thank the following individuals for their participation in the review of this report: Sarah Brown, National Campaign to Prevent Teenage Pregnancy, Washington, DC; Michael I. Cohen, Department of Pediatrics, Albert Einstein College of Medicine; Elizabeth McAnarney, Department of Pediatrics, University of Rochester Medical Center; Elena Nightingale, Scholar-in-Residence, National Research Council; Jack P. Shonkoff, Graduate School for Advanced Studies in Social Welfare, Brandeis University; and Ruby Takanishi, Foundation for Child Development, New York, NY.

Although the individuals listed above have provided constructive comments and suggestions, it must be emphasized that responsibility for this final report rests entirely with the authoring committee and the institution.

We hope this report will stimulate and encourage researchers, service providers, and policy makers to search for new ways to ensure that all adolescents grow to become healthy, happy, and productive adults.

David A. Hamburg, *Chair*
Michele D. Kipke, *Director*
Forum on Adolescence

Adolescent Development and the Biology of Puberty

Adolescence is one of the most fascinating and complex transitions in the life span. Its breathtaking pace of growth and change is second only to that of infancy. Biological processes drive many aspects of this growth and development, with the onset of puberty marking the passage from childhood to adolescence. Puberty is a transitional period between childhood and adulthood, during which a growth spurt occurs, secondary sexual characteristics appear, fertility is achieved, and profound psychological changes take place.

Although the sequence of pubertal changes is relatively predictable, their timing is extremely variable. The normal range of onset is ages 8 to 14 in females and ages 9 to 15 in males, with girls generally experiencing physiological growth characteristic of the onset of puberty two years before boys. Pubertal maturation is controlled largely by complex interactions among the brain, the pituitary gland, and the gonads, which in turn interact with environment (i.e., the social, cultural, and ambient environment). A relatively new area of research related to puberty is that of brain development. Evidence now suggests that brain growth continues into adolescence, including the proliferation of the support cells, which nourish the neurons, and myelination, which permits faster neural processing. These changes in the brain are likely to stimulate cognitive growth and development, including the capacity for abstract reasoning.

Although the biology of physical growth and maturation during puberty is generally understood, available data on the biochemical and physiological mediators of human behavior are extremely primitive, and their clinical applicability remains obscure. Despite the limitations of available data, a substantial body of evidence suggests that variations in the age of onset of puberty may have developmental and behavioral consequences during adolescence. Mounting evidence also suggests that gonadal hormones, gonadotropins, and adrenal hormones influence and are affected by social interactions among groups of experimental animals, and they may also play an important role in regulating human social behavior. Interesting and potentially informative parallels exist between the maturational process in human beings and in other animals, especially those having well-documented social structures.

Research conducted with both humans and nonhuman primates suggests that adolescence is a time for carrying out crucial developmental tasks: becoming physically and sexually mature; acquiring skills needed to carry out adult roles; gaining increased autonomy from parents; and realigning social ties with members of both the same and the opposite gender. Studies of such commonalities underscore the critical importance of this part of the life course in establishing social skills. For many social species, such skills are further developed through peer-oriented interactions that are distinct from both earlier child-adult patterns and later adult pairings.

Adolescence is a time of tremendous growth and potential, but it is also a time of considerable risk. Most people would argue that being an adolescent today is a different experience from what it was even a few decades ago. Both the perceptions of this change and the change itself attest to the powerful influence of social contexts on adolescent development. Many of the 34 million adolescents in the United States are confronting pressures to use alcohol, cigarettes, or other drugs and to initiate sexual relationships at earlier ages, putting themselves at high risk for intentional and unintentional injuries, unintended pregnancies, and infection from sexually transmitted diseases (STDs), including the human immunodeficiency virus (HIV). Many experience a wide range of painful and debilitating mental health problems.

One of the important insights to emerge from scientific inquiry into adolescence in the past decade is the profound influence of settings on adolescents' behavior and development. Until recently, research conducted to understand adolescent behavior, particularly risk-related behaviors, focused on the individual characteristics of teenagers and their families. In 1993, the National Research Council conducted a study that took a critical look at how families, communities, and other institutions are serving the needs of youth in the United States. This study concluded that adolescents depend not only on their families, but also on the neighborhoods in which they live, the schools that they attend, the health care system, and the workplace from which they learn a wide range of important skills. If sufficiently enriched, all of these settings and social institutions in concert can help teenagers successfully make the transition from childhood to adulthood.

Family income is perhaps the single most important factor in determining the settings in which adolescents spend their lives. Housing, neighborhoods, schools, and the social opportunities that are linked to them are largely controlled by income; a family's income and employment status decide its access to health care services and strongly influence the quality of those services (National Research Council, 1993). Opportunities for advanced education and training and entry into the workforce are also closely linked to family income. Moreover, income is a powerful influence in shaping what is arguably the most important setting, the family. At this point in time, the evidence is clear—persistent poverty exacts a significant price on adolescents' health, development, educational attainment, and socioeconomic potential, even though the causal relationships are not well understood in all cases.

Not only is current research attempting to more fully characterize the physiological mechanisms responsible for initiating and regulating neuroendocrine maturation and somatic growth, but it is also attempting to characterize these environmental and contextual factors that may interact with biological ones to enhance or impede maturation. This research is attempting to address questions that could help to inform the development of policies and the delivery of services for youth. Such questions include: What is the pubertal experience like for teenagers today, and how does it differ from that in the past, both in the United States and in other cultures? How do pubertal experiences, in some circumstances and for some subgroups, trigger maladaptive responses? What role do pubertal processes play in cognitive change? How does puberty, in conjunction with other events that occur during early adolescence, influence the emergence of developmental psychopathology?

CHANGES IN THE STUDY OF ADOLESCENT DEVELOPMENT

Over the last two decades, the research base in the field of adolescent development has undergone a growth spurt. Knowledge has expanded significantly. New studies have allowed more complex views of the multiple dimensions of adolescence, fresh insights into the process and timing of puberty, and new perspectives on the behaviors associated with the second decade of life. At the same time, the field's underlying theoretical assumptions have changed and matured.

Researchers of human development have consistently observed that the second decade of life is a time of dramatic change: a period of rapid physical growth, endocrine (hormone) changes, cognitive development and increasing analytic capability; emotional growth, a time of self-exploration and increasing independence, and active participation in a more complex social universe. For much of this century, scientists and scholars studying adolescence tended to assume that the changes associated with adolescence were almost entirely dictated by biological influences. It has been viewed as a time of storm and stress, best contained or passed through as quickly as possible. *Adolescence*, a 1904 book by G. Stanley Hall, typified this standpoint. It was Hall who popularized the notion that adolescence is inevitably a time of psychological and emotional turmoil (Hall, 1904). Half a century later, psychoanalytic writers including Anna Freud accepted and augmented Hall's emphasis on turmoil (Petersen, 1988). Even today, "raging hormones" continue to be a popular explanation for the lability, aggression, and sexual activity associated with adolescence (Litt, 1995). Intense conflict between adolescents and their parents is often considered an unavoidable consequence of adolescence (Petersen, 1988). However, this assumption is not supported by scientific evidence. The assumption that turmoil and conflict are inevitable consequences of the teenage years may even have prevented some adolescents from receiving the support and services they needed.

Research is now creating a more realistic view of adolescence. Adolescence continues to be seen as a period of time encompassing difficult developmental challenges, but there is wider recognition that biology is only one factor that affects young people's development, adjustment, and behavior. In fact, there is mounting evidence that parents, members of the community, service providers, and social institutions can both promote healthy development among adolescents and intervene effectively when problems arise.

The study of adolescence is now becoming an increasingly sophisticated science. Thanks to powerful new research tools and other scientific and technological advances, today's theories of adolescent development are more likely to be supported by scientific evidence than in the past. Indeed, there has been sufficient research to allow a reassessment of the nature of adolescent development. At the same time, there is greater recognition that neither puberty nor adolescence can be understood without considering the social and cultural contexts in which young people grow and develop, including the familial and societal values, social and economic conditions, and institutions that they experience. This research has contributed the following to our understanding of adolescence:

The adolescent years need not be troubled years. There is now greater recognition that young people can move through the adolescent years without experiencing great trauma or getting into serious trouble; most young people do. Although adolescence can certainly be a challenging span of years, individuals negotiate it with varying degrees of difficulty, just as they do other periods of life. Moreover, when problems do arise during adolescence they should not be considered as "normal"—i.e., that the adolescent will grow out of it—nor should they be ignored (Petersen, 1988).

Only a segment of the adolescent population is at high risk for experiencing serious problems. Over the past 50 years, studies conducted in North America and Europe have documented that only about a quarter of the adolescent population is at high risk for, or more vulnerable to, a wide range of psychosocial problems (Carnegie Corporation of New York, 1995). These adolescents are not believed to be at increased risk because of biological or hormonal changes associated with puberty, but rather from a complex interaction among biological, environmental, and social factors. Indeed, as discussed by Anne Petersen, there is mounting evidence that most biological changes interact with a wide range of contextual, psychological, social, and environmental factors that affect behavior (Buchanan et al., 1992; Susman, 1997, see also Brooks-Gunn et al., 1994). Researchers are also concluding that behaviors associated with adolescence, including some high-risk behaviors, are influenced by the social milieu (Brooks-Gunn and Reiter, 1990). Studies show that, in contrast to children and adults, the most common causes of mortality among adolescents are associated with social, environmental, and behavioral factors rather than genetic, congenital, or biological diseases. Indeed, many of today's adolescents are using alcohol and other drugs, engaging in unprotected sexual intercourse, and are both victims and perpetrators of violence, which puts them at increased risk for a wide range of developmental and health-related problems, including morbidity and mortality. It is important to note that the leading causes of morbidity and mortality among adolescents are entirely preventable. Although relatively small, a significant number of adolescents also experience morbidity and mortality associated with genetic and congenital disorders (such as cystic fibrosis, muscular dystrophy, cerebral palsy), cancer, and infectious diseases that affect their development, behavior, and well-being.

Adolescent behavior is influenced by complex interactions between the biological and social contexts. In the past, researchers tended to conduct research designed to examine the impact of hormones on adolescent behavior. While this work continues, there is now an appreciation for the complex reciprocal relationship and interaction between biological and social environments, and the interaction between these environments and adolescent behavior (Graber et al., 1997).

Current understanding of adolescent development remains limited. Although the study of adolescence is becoming more sophisticated in nature, researchers also recognize that the current knowledge base on adolescent development and behavior is quite limited. The research conducted to date has predominately been descriptive in nature, relied on cross-sectional data, and been unidimensional in focus. Indeed, few research studies have successfully considered the multiple factors that collectively influence adolescent development. As discussed by Iris Litt, there is now a growing appreciation that new research is needed, including research that employs longitudinal designs; characterizes developmental changes associated with the onset of puberty well before the age of 8; and seeks to characterize growth and development across the life span—i.e., from infancy to adolescence, young adulthood, adulthood, and the senior years. Studying these developmental stages in isolation from one another provides only a partial and incomplete picture.

Researchers from diverse fields, including the biological, behavioral, and social sciences, have developed new techniques to study adolescent development. Use of more rigorous research methods has improved the reliability and validity of the measurement techniques used, and consequently the ability to document the multifaceted dimensions of growth and maturation during adolescence. For example, the development of radioimmunoassay methodology in the late 1960s, and the considerable refinement of that process over the decades, have made it possible to study the hormones that control reproductive maturation. The development of neuroimaging technology in the 1970s created exciting new opportunities for studying brain development; these techniques include more sensitive, easy-to-use hormone assay technology and new brain imaging technologies, allowing insight into brain development and function. Moreover, longitudinal studies are increasingly being designed to characterize the interaction among genetic, biological, familial, environmental, social, and behavioral factors (both risk and protective in nature) among children and adolescents. For example, a valuable new source of data that has the potential to significantly advance the knowledge base of physiological and behavioral development among adolescents is the National Longitudinal Study of Adolescent Health (called Add Health). From the collection of longitudinal data, it will be possible to examine how the timing and tempo of puberty influences social and cognitive development among teenagers. This dataset will also permit analyses to examine how family-, school- and individual-level risk and protective factors are associated with adolescent health and morbidity (e.g., emotional health, violence, substance use, sexuality).

An increasing number of disciplines are beginning to conduct research on adolescent development. Understanding adolescent development requires answers to a number of difficult questions: how do adolescents develop physically, how do their relationships with parents and friends change, how are young people as a group viewed and treated by society, how does adolescence in our society differ from adolescence in other cultures, and how has adolescence and adolescent development changed over the past few decades. A complete understanding of adolescence, and the potential to answer these questions depends on an integrated approach, and involvement of a wide range of disciplines, including but not limited to endocrinology, psychology, sociology, psychiatry, genetics, anthropology, neuroscience, history, and economics. While each discipline offers its own view point regarding adolescence and adolescent development, the field will not be able to successfully answer these questions without integrating the contributions of different disciplines into a coherent and comprehensive viewpoint. Fortunately, studies of puberty are increasingly drawing on and therefore benefiting from the knowledge base of these diverse fields.

KEY FINDINGS OF RECENT STUDIES

The workshop included a series of panel discussions that focused on adolescence as experienced by both human and nonhuman primates, including neuroendocrine physiology at puberty, the interplay between pubertal development and behavior, and implications for research, policy, and practice. Here we briefly summarize key findings from some of the studies that were discussed at the workshop (also see Crockett and Petersen, 1993; Grumbach and Styne, 1998; Pusey, 1990; Suomi, 1997;1991). As previously noted, this summary is not intended to provide a comprehensive review of the new research in this field; rather, it highlights important new findings that emerged during the workshop presentations and discussions.

In the United States, the onset of puberty occurs earlier than was previously recognized. Over the last 150 years, girls' sexual maturation, as measured by the age of menarche, is occurring at younger ages in all developed countries by at least two to three years. In the mid-nineteenth century, the average age at which girls reached menarche was approximately 15. The trend toward earlier menarche is now being documented in developing countries as well. Improved diets and more effective public health measures are the reasons often cited for this trend (Garn, 1992).

Research conducted during the 1990s greatly enhanced researchers' understanding of the age of puberty among girls. For example, although the onset of menarche is still considered to be a significant indicator of the tempo of maturation, researchers now view menarche as a late event in the pubertal process. At the workshop, Frank Biro presented data from the Growth and Health Study funded by the National Heart, Lung, and Blood Institute. This longitudinal study enrolled a cohort of over 2,000 girls, ages 9 to 10 years in 1987-1988; approximately half of the sample was white and half was black; the sample was recruited from clinics at three clinical centers located in Richmond, California, Cincinnati, Ohio, and metropolitan Washington, D.C. According to the study design, girls' maturation stage and body mass index were assessed annually; data for other variables, such as household income, nutrition, physical activity, cardiovascular risk factors, self-esteem and self-perception, and other psychosocial measures, were collected biennially (Brown et al., 1998). Almost half of the participants had begun puberty before the onset of the study. According to Biro, indicators of pubertal growth have been observed as early as age 7. These findings suggest that as children experience puberty and other developmental changes at earlier ages, there may be the need to consider how to design and deliver age-appropriate interventions during the middle childhood and preteen years, to help them avoid harmful or risky behaviors and develop a health-promoting lifestyle.

There is significant variation among individuals in the timing of puberty. There is variation in both the onset and the tempo of puberty. Research shows that the timing of puberty can affect other aspects of development, especially for girls. Jeanne Brooks-Gunn discussed the findings from a recent study, which recruited a community sample of nearly 2,000 high school students from urban and rural areas of western Oregon. The study found that early-maturing girls and late-maturing boys showed more evidence of adjustment problems than other adolescents (Graber et al., 1997).

Multiple factors affect the age of puberty. Research now suggests that the timing of puberty can be affected by a wide range of factors, including genetic and biological influences, stress and stressful life events, socioeconomic status, environmental toxins, nutrition and diet, exercise, amount of fat and body weight, and the presence of a chronic illness. Research also shows that the family, the peer group, the neighborhood, the school, the workplace, and the broader society have all been shown to influence adolescent developmental outcomes, although it is less clear if these factors influence pubertal development. With respect to school settings, research suggests that the transition from small elementary schools to larger, more anonymous middle schools can be a stressful event in the lives of children (National Research Council, 1993). Some of the stressful influences or events factors mentioned above have been correlated with pubertal timing, but a causal relationship cannot be assumed.

Stress does not trigger puberty, but it does modulate the timing of puberty. In her remarks at the workshop, Elizabeth Susman took note of research correlating stress and the timing of puberty.[1] A review of this literature shows that researchers observe different effects of stress at differ-

---

[1] For the purposes of this discussion, stress is defined as a physical, mental, or emotional strain or tension. Stress is a normal part of everyone's life and need not be either good or bad; reactions to stress however, can vary considerably, with some reactions being unpleasant and/or undesirable.

ent stages of puberty (Susman et al., 1989). For example, stress appears to delay maturation for young adolescents but to precipitate puberty for older adolescents. According to Susman, it makes sense that stress would delay maturation because stress hormones tend to suppress reproductive hormones (Susman, 1997; Graber and Warren, 1992). She added that her research has not yet resolved the question of directionality: Do environmental stressors affect the reproductive hormones, or does the rate of maturation affect the level of circulating stress hormones? Other participants at the meeting noted that social factors influence this process as well. For example, family conflict appears to be associated with earlier menarche in girls (Graber et al., 1995).

There is some evidence that, on average, girls experience more distress during adolescence than boys. Some researchers have speculated that, for girls, the transition during puberty brings about greater vulnerability to other environmental stressors (Ge et al., 1995). In particular, a growing literature suggests that the early onset of puberty can have an adverse effect on girls' development (Caspi et al., 1993; Ge et al., 1996). It can affect their physical development (they tend to be shorter and heavier), their behavior (they have higher rates of conduct disorders); and emotional development (they tend to have lower self-esteem and higher rates of depression, eating disorders, and suicide). The youngest, most mature children are those at greatest risk for delinquency.

Early-maturing boys also appear to have higher rates of delinquency (Graber et al., 1997; Rutter and Smith, 1995). Generally speaking, however, boys who mature early fare better than late bloomers. Because they are taller and more muscular than their age-mates, they may be more confident, more popular, and more successful both in the classroom and on the playing field. In contrast, late-maturing boys have a poorer self-image, poorer school performance, and lower educational aspirations and expectations (Dorn et al., 1988; Litt, 1995).

Girls from ethnic minority groups may be reaching puberty earlier than white girls. Data presented at the workshop show that for black girls, the average age of menarche is 12.1 years, compared with 12.9 years for white girls (see Brown et al., 1998). Black girls also begin pubertal development earlier than their white peers do—by 15 months. Interestingly, even though they reach menarche earlier, tempo of the pubertal development is slower. Researchers have also found that self-esteem does not follow the same developmental pattern in black and white girls. It appears that black girls' higher self-esteem may be rooted in cultural differences in attitudes toward physical appearance and obesity (Brown et al., 1998). In general, however, the factors that protect some girls and place others at risk are not well understood. It is important to note that these findings are preliminary in nature, and more research is need to further validate them, as well as determine if these differences apply to girls from other ethnic, and racial groups, such as Hispanics, American Indians, Asians, and Pacific Islanders.

Puberty may be a better predictor of aggression and problem behaviors than age. There is growing evidence to suggest that puberty rather than chronological age may signal the onset of delinquency and problem behaviors among some teenagers (Keenan and Shaw, 1997; Rutter et al., 1998). For example, early maturers—both male and female—are more likely than other adolescents to report delinquency. Early-maturing females also appear to be at increased risk for victimization, especially sexual assault, and this may partially explain their greater likelihood of problem behaviors (Flannery et al., 1993; Raine et al., 1997). These findings suggest the need for interventions that are targeted to early-maturing adolescents who may be at increased risk for a wide range of behavior problems and associated poor developmental outcomes.

Physical maturation appears to have little correlation with cognitive development. Many developmental psychologists, most notably Jean Piaget, have documented an expanded capacity for abstract reasoning during adolescence. Today's adolescents are often capable of complex reasoning and moral judgment; their capacities frequently astonish parents and teachers. Indeed, IQ tests show an overall gain in cognitive capacities since the 1940s, when military personnel were tested in large numbers and achieved a median score of about 100. However, there appears to be little relationship between physical and cognitive maturation.

Researchers have tested the hypothesis that growth across the developmental spectrum—physical, cognitive, social, and emotional—proceeds on a similar timetable, and they have found little evidence to support this hypothesis. However, the research in this area is relatively weak, in part due to a lack of reliable, valid, easily administered instruments for assessing cognitive development (Litt, 1995). When cognitive development and capacities are not in sync with physical and sexual maturation, young people are more vulnerable; this also creates special challenges for designing and delivering age appropriate clinical interventions and services. Adults will often assume that adolescents who look older have a better grasp of the consequences of their actions.

Brain development appears to continue during adolescence. One of most remarkable findings in neurobiology over the last decade is the extent of change that can occur in the brain, even in the adult brain, as a function of the physical, social, and intellectual environment.

Starting in infancy and continuing into later childhood, there is a period of exuberant synapse growth followed by a period of synaptic "pruning" which is largely completed by puberty. Although, neuroscientists have documented the time line of this synaptic waxing and waning, they are less sure about what it means for changes in childrens' and adolescents' cognitive development, behavior, intelligence, and capacity to learn. Generally, they point to correlations between changes in synaptic density or numbers and observed changes in behavior based on developmental and cognitive psychology. In coming decades, research tools such as positron emission tomography (PET) scans and functional magnetic resonance imaging (MRI) scans should greatly expand researchers' knowledge about adolescent brain development. In particular, functional imaging, if repeated over time, carries the potential for providing a better understanding of the functional connections between brain development and psychological performance (including cognitive development). New insights into brain development may also shed light on some psychopathologies and learning disabilities that affect preteens and adolescents, such as attention deficit/ hyperactivity disorder (ADHD), depressive disorders, and schizophrenia.

Researchers are also providing new insights into the relationship between gender, hormones, brain development, and behavior. In terms of the onset of puberty, boys generally follow girls by two years. For example, boys typically reach their maximum height velocity two years later than girls. In the realm of neuroscience, there is new evidence of divergent patterns of male and female brain development; these patterns have been observed between the ages of 5 and 7. Case in point: during this period, the amygdala (a part of the limbic system concerned with the expression and regulation of emotion and motivation) increases robustly in males, but not in females; the hippocampus (a part of the limbic system that plays an important role in organizing memories) increases robustly in females, but not in males. The basal ganglia are larger in females; this appears to be significant, since boys are more likely to have disorders, such as ADHD, that are associated with smaller basal ganglia. Girls may have extra protection against this type of disorder. Although there are clear differences in the path of brain development for girls and boys, it is not yet possible to look at a brain scan and determine whether the subject is male or female.

Pregnancy during adolescence may alter the physiological development of girls. During pregnancy, young women at different points in pubertal development show comparable hormone profiles. Pregnancy in very young women may compromise their skeletal growth, preventing them from reaching maximum bone mass. Frank Biro noted that his research team, which followed several hundred adolescent pregnancies, found that, after giving birth, adolescent mothers were on average significantly heavier (by approximately 10 pounds) and fatter (having thicker skin folds) than their counterparts who had not given birth.

RESEARCH CHALLENGES

The final session of the workshop focused on a broad view of the field of puberty and adolescent development, considering the implications of recent advances for the future of research, as well as its effects on current policies and practices. Summarizing the comments made by workshop participants, we outline below a number of challenges that researchers now face in moving this area of inquiry to its next stage of development. Gaps within the current knowledge base of adolescent development that require further research as identified by the presenters are also summarized.

Adolescence should be recognized as a credible area of scientific inquiry. Numerous workshop participants emphasized the need to build the capacity of the field of adolescent research with new funding for longitudinal research and incentives for providing professional training and conducting interdisciplinary research.

The many studies showing that adolescence is not necessarily a time of storm and stress (Elkind, 1992; Hamburg, 1992) represent a significant shift in perspective. However, there has been relatively little research on the affective and attitudinal characteristics often associated with the adolescent period—elation, thrill seeking, excitement, moodiness, shifts in energy, irritability, restlessness. Only recently have studies linked negative emotional or affective states to the hormonal changes of puberty, particularly in normal children (Buchanan et al., 1992).

Advancing the field's understanding of adolescence requires a focus on research and on the policies that are ideally informed by this research. Existing theoretical models should be expanded to take advantage of advances in the biomedical sciences. As workshop participant Elizabeth Susman observed, "Further integration of physiological processes into models of adolescent development will enable scientists to construct more holistic, integrative models than currently are available" (Susman, 1997).

Research is needed to explore the relationship among various aspects of pubertal growth by creating and applying more complex modeling procedures. Until quite recently, models of adolescent development tended to be unidirectional, allowing researchers to track either behavior or hormones. Some progress was then made in developing bidirectional analyses, showing the interaction between behavior and hormones. Only recently have investigators looked seriously at physical and social factors that may influence adolescent development. Consequently, existing models do not afford the opportunity to take more than a snapshot of adolescence or, at best, to conduct longitudinal studies that follow the trajectory of one or another variable. Advances in the understanding of adolescence therefore hinge on the development of more complex, multidimensional theoretical and statistical models—i.e., a "global weather map" of puberty. An interdisciplinary effort is needed to develop such models.

Research is needed to further study the age of onset of menarche and differences among girls of different racial and ethnic groups. According to some researchers, "maturational timing appears to be the same across ethnic groups, provided nutrition is adequate" (Brooks-Gunn and Reiter, 1990). As they acknowledge, however, this assertion is controversial within the field, and many questions remain.

In light of research that suggests that black girls reach menarche earlier than white girls, which factors contribute to the early onset of puberty for black girls? Can we assume that the reasons for differences in the timing of menarche are the same today as they were in the 1960s? If, as discussed earlier, black girls begin puberty approximately 15 months before their white counterparts, but they arrive at menarche only 8 months earlier, what accounts for their slower tempo of pubertal development? What is the relationship between body weight and age of puberty for black and white girls? Do girls who are heavier have a slower tempo of pubertal development? How important are different cultural attitudes toward body image? What insights might cross-cultural studies provide?

Although much of the current research focuses on the different course of puberty among black and white girls, clearly there is a need for additional research to characterize differences in the timing of puberty and menarche (and outcomes associated with these differences) in an increasingly racially and ethnically diverse adolescent population in the United States. This research must go beyond black-white comparisons to other racial and ethnic groups, such as Hispanics, American Indians, and Asians and Pacific Islanders. Moreover, given the heterogeneity that exists within these groups, within-group comparisons are also needed—e.g., comparisons of African Americans, Nigerians, and Caribbean blacks within black populations; Cubans, Puerto Ricans, Central Americans, and Mexicans within Hispanic populations; and Chinese, Japanese, and Vietnamese within Asian populations. How do genetic and cultural factors affect the timing of pubertal development and the timing of menarche? An anthropologist taking part in the workshop noted that, among the Lumi people of New Guinea, the average age of menarche is significantly later than it is in the United States and other developed countries.

Research is needed to investigate the relationship between adrenarche and puberty. Puberty is now considered to be one event along a continuum of development. It is preceded by adrenarche (the reinitiating of adrenal androgen secretion), which begins about two years before what has traditionally been considered the onset of puberty. Heredity appears to play a major role in determining the onset of adrenarche as well as puberty. Adrenarche is still poorly understood; its function is not entirely clear. Researchers initially thought that adrenarche causes a prepubertal growth spurt between the ages of 5 and 7, but it is difficult to attribute this "blip" to adrenarche, since adrenal androgen secretion continues while growth drops back to its former rate. Are there cross-cultural and cross-national differences with respect to the onset of adrenarche? If so, why?

Research is needed to explore further the relationship between sex steroids and behavior. It is commonly thought that pubertal change affects moods and behavior, but the evidence is mixed (Richards and Larson, 1993). Despite decades of speculation, the effects of sex steroids, in particular on moods and behavior, during adolescence remain unclear. What is the relationship between the adrenal and gonadal systems (or HPA and HPG systems) and their influence on mood and behavior? Many researchers are looking at these relationships, but more research is needed. Reliable and valid measures that will permit examinations with greater specificity are needed to determine how the pubertal rise in hormone concentrations affects cognition, as well as its effect on problem behaviors, such as aggression.

Research is needed to study vulnerability and resiliency across the spectrum of child and adolescent development. Why are some preteens and adolescents more or less vulnerable or resilient given comparable life events and contexts in which they are growing and developing? Are biological systems more or less sensitive to life events and contexts at certain points in time? If so, do genetic influences predispose some youth to be more or less vulnerable, or conversely, more or less resilient? For example, if an adolescent girl develops an eating disorder, does her life trajectory in general, and the biological impact of the disease in particular, depend on the point in her development when it occurs?

Research is needed to study the factors that promote or impede cognitive development in adolescence. The field would benefit from a more complex model of adolescent cognitive development. Why does cognitive development proceed on a different timetable than physical and sexual maturation? Researchers focusing on puberty have not detected the effects of steroids on cognitive functioning, but, in menopause, estrogen therapy demonstrably affects cognitive functioning. What accounts for this discrepancy? How is the architecture of the brain related to adolescent cognitive development? Will functional MRI studies enhance knowledge in this area? Moreover, we need to better understand the decision-making processes of adolescents and the factors that motivate them to engage in high-risk versus health promoting behaviors.

Research is needed to expand the field's understanding of the effects of stress—both negative and positive forms of stress—on adolescent development. Researchers have just recently begun to establish a connection between stress and the timing of pubertal maturation. New research is needed to identify adverse environmental conditions (such as those associated with poverty) that may affect the long-term suppression or stimulation of endocrine processes that, in turn, may affect normal growth and psychological development (Susman, 1997).

Research is needed to further clarify developmental differences according to gender. Why do girls reach puberty before boys? What are the implications with respect to health promotion and the prevention of risky behaviors? What are the implications of gender differences in brain development?

Research is needed to address key issues in adolescent development in light of advances in genetics. Adolescence is a time when a whole set of genetic influences become more important while another set of genetic factors, which were apparent in early life, become less important. For example, there is clear evidence for a genetic predisposition to schizophrenia, and the onset of schizophrenia typically occurs during the later adolescent years. What interaction between the host and environment signals the onset of schizophrenia during adolescence? Can we with greater specificity account for how and when these as well as other genetic "signals" are turned on or off during childhood as well as adolescence? How are new genetic mechanisms brought into play? What are the factors, both genetic and nongenetic, that can influence the expression of specific genes during adolescence? Increasing knowledge about the interaction of multiple genes, the environment, and behavior will someday help to inform the development of new strategies to promote the healthy development of both children and adolescents.

In summary, as discussed at the workshop, there are a number of challenges for conducting research in this area, as well as clear opportunities for advancing the knowledge base regarding adolescent development, health, behavior, and well-being. The next generation of research studies needs to be interdisciplinary in nature; to integrate cross-sectional and longitudinal research methods with more sophisticated modeling techniques to examine the interrelationship among genetic, biological, social, and environmental influences and their unique and shared contribution to adolescent development; and to be couched within a broader developmental framework.

POLICY CHALLENGES

In discussing the state of research on puberty and adolescent development, workshop participants turned to issues related to policy and practice.

Summarizing their remarks, we outline below some opportunities to inform policy and practice through scientific research.

The gap among research, policy, and practice needs to be narrowed. As in many other fields of science, in the field of adolescent development more knowledge is available than is put to use. Although there is much more still to learn, the knowledge base is already sufficient to allow reconsideration of many policies now. The communication of research findings to policy makers, service providers, educators, parents, and young people may help them develop more effective strategies for addressing the opportunities and challenges of adolescence, including helping adolescents to learn how to form close, durable human relationships; feel a sense of worth as a person; express constructive curiosity and exploratory behavior; know how to use the support systems available to them; succeed at school; and acquire the technical and analytic capabilities to participate in a world-class economy (Carnegie Corporation of New York, 1995). In particular, parents, educators, health providers, and human service providers need to have a greater awareness that puberty begins earlier than most people imagine (especially for girls), that early-maturing girls may be at higher risk for depression and problem behaviors, that many factors affect the timing and course of pubertal development, and that physical or sexual maturation is most likely on a different schedule than cognitive development. Finally, individuals or groups that make decisions about important legal and social questions need access to such information so they can make the kinds of decisions that protect the health and well-being of youth. For example, research findings should be used to undergird policies and regulations regarding when it is appropriate for adolescents to be treated as adults—by courts, health agencies, sex education programs, and schools.

Research needs to be applied to promote positive developmental outcomes. Studies of the timing of puberty suggest that preventive efforts need to start earlier—particularly interventions designed to prevent problem behaviors, such as violence. Research findings can help policy makers determine when particular interventions are most likely to be effective, and for whom. One workshop participant pointed out that, too often, conduct disorders are not identified until a child reaches adolescence. As the knowledge base expands, it may become more possible to recognize, in advance of puberty, which children are at risk for such disorders and to provide anticipatory guidance. Research can also point to subpopulations (such as children born to adolescent mothers) that may be more likely to encounter problems in adolescence (Hardy et al., 1997; Graber and Brooks-Gunn, 1999). A key challenge is to track and anticipate different patterns of maturation before they actually occur and to encourage parents, teachers, health care providers, and other key players to provide primary prevention intervention.

The focus needs to shift to one that embraces both prevention and health promotion. A shift in emphasis is needed from simply preventing problems to actively promoting a wide range of healthful behaviors. Policy makers and practitioners need the kind of information that will help them promote healthy development, including information about what is happening at various stages of adolescence; how hormonal changes interact with contextual factors and how they affect sexual arousal; and the risk factors affecting early, middle, and late maturers. For example, preventing unwanted pregnancy and infection with STDs is an urgent concern for all those who raise adolescents or who work with them. Some ethnic or cultural groups look favorably on early marriage and childbirth and, within these groups, young mothers and their children tend to fare well. However, across the United States, most teenage pregnancies are unplanned and unwanted. Fortunately, the nation has made some progress in reducing rates of unintended pregnancies among teenagers in recent years (Institute of Medicine, 1995). After reaching 117 pregnancies per 1000 females ages 15-19 in 1990, the pregnancy rate has fallen a total of 17 percent between 1990 and 1996 to 97 births per 1000 females ages 15-19; these pregnancy data include births, abortions, and miscarriages (Henshaw, 1998). Despite these improvements, these rates remain high thus warranting further attention. Research shows that other nations are doing much better at ensuring the health and well-being of adolescents and helping them avert unwanted pregnancies. Young people in other countries have similar patterns of sexual activity; however, they have access to better information and supports, including sex education and contraception.

Resources need to be invested in an effort to promote sound decision making among adolescents. Adolescents are capable of impressive intellectual feats, but research shows that studies of cognitive capacity in artificial settings (such as laboratories and classrooms) may overestimate what adolescents are able to do in real life, in which stress and time pressure are often intense (Petersen and Leffert, in press). Moreover, a wide range of factors, such as social coercion and the use of alcohol and other drugs may influence and compromise adolescents' ability to accurately process information to make well-informed choices. For this reason, it is often useful to distinguish between the kind of "cold cognition" described by cognitive scientists—formal operations, the capacity for abstract thought— and "hot cognition"—the capacity to reason and make multiple decisions under conditions of high anxiety and stress. Too little is known about hot cognition. It is clear, however, that adolescents need more help in coping with the kinds of situations in which competent decision making is essential.

Cross-cultural studies raise key questions. What insights can be drawn from studies of other countries, in which youth are engaging in fewer high-risk behaviors? Are adolescents in the United States engaging in risky behaviors because they have had too few opportunities to learn how to avoid them and make good decisions? Is there a need for more and better models of responsible adult decision making, both in their communities and in the media? Many other cultures expect youth to take on adult roles earlier, and they lay the groundwork for adult decision making. What kind of policies or programs will strengthen adolescents' capacity for sound decision making? What are the mechanisms underlying changes in cognitive capacities, leading toward adult intellectual functioning? What kinds of experiences and tools can be provided to adolescents that will help them learn to make good decisions? What kinds of settings and experiences will further their moral development?

Cultural diversity must be taken into account when studying adolescence and planning interventions. In efforts to understand adolescence and promote good outcomes for young people and their families, the importance of cultural context cannot be overstated. The same conditions or circumstances may pose different risks and challenges for different groups. For example, different cultures have different attitudes toward sexual precocity and sexual behavior, including early pregnancy and childrearing. Early puberty poses fewer problems for girls in cultures whose adult women tend to support early maturation; for example, there is limited research suggesting that black girls cope better with early maturation than their white peers. Clearly this research needs to be further replicated, conducted with both girls and boys, and conducted with a diverse group of teens—i.e., with teenagers from a variety of racial and ethnic groups.

These findings have important implications for professionals who work with adolescents and their parents. Not every early-maturing girl is at high risk. Moreover, research shows that adolescents growing up in different contexts may have different views of their own development. White girls may be more likely than black or Hispanic girls to value a thin body type; they are more likely to restrict their diets and to smoke, affecting their pubertal development. Studies also indicate that young people from different ethnic or cultural groups tend to have different estimations of their own physical and sexual maturity, regardless of the objective evidence.

Adolescents should be included in efforts intended to improve outcomes for them and their families. Given access to good schools, access to preventive information, needed services, and strong social supports, young people can control their own behavior through effective cognitive, self-regulatory, and self-management techniques. They can learn to respond to stressful life events and the unpredictable nature of day-to-day life as experienced by most adolescents and adults. They can also serve as positive role models within their schools and communities and encourage their peers to engage in health promoting behaviors.

In summary, as discussed at the workshop, there are a number of opportunities to inform policy through research. Specifically, participants discussed the need to construct policies and design programs that focus on both prevention and health promotion; that seek to promote positive developmental outcomes (not just the absence of problems); that engage adolescents as young adults (rather than talking down to them as if they were children). Moreover, in light of the growing diversity in the adolescent population, policies must ensure that health care and social services are delivered in a culturally relevant and sensitive manner.

IMPROVING PUBLIC UNDERSTANDING

In the course of the workshop discussions, participants identified a number of important findings from research that should be communicated to increase the public's understanding of the reality of adolescence. Summarizing the comments of workshop participants, we lay out below some of the most important messages that can be communicated to parents, teachers, health care providers, and others who live and work with adolescents.

Sexually transmitted diseases and other health problems pose a major threat to adolescents. It is clear, from nearly three decades of research, that adolescents are at high risk for infection with STDs, including HIV; rates of infection with STDs are higher among adolescents and young adults than any other age group, and incidence rates of HIV infection remain alarmingly high among teenagers (Institute of Medicine, 1995). All adolescents require the knowledge and skills needed to protect themselves from STDs, HIV, and unintended pregnancy. There remains the need to deliver effective prevention and health promotion interventions to all adolescents, to ensure that they have long, productive, and healthy lives. The public can play a very important role to ensure the health, safety, security, and well-being of adolescents. For example, health providers and educators can and should provide adolescents with the knowledge and skills they require to protect themselves from a wide range of public health problems, including STDs, HIV, alcohol and other drug abuse, and violence. Parents can also play an important role by encouraging and facilitating meaningful discussions with their teenagers in an effort to provide them with needed information and skills, as well as to provide them with the opportunity to explore their own values and beliefs. Finally, the media can play a very important role by reinforcing prevention and health promotion messages.

Children need health monitoring and care during the elementary and middle school years. Puberty begins earlier than most parents and many health professionals realize. And yet, many 5- to 11-year-olds are rarely seen in doctors' offices or health centers unless they have an acute health care need or a serious medical problem. Once the well-baby visits of infancy and toddlerhood are over and a full round of immunizations has been completed, most parents seldom take their children to the doctor. As a result, parents lack the kind of information and guidance they need to help them fully understand and appreciate the developmental changes experienced by the prepubescent child. Some problems that could be addressed in middle childhood (including growth problems and behavioral issues) may go unrecognized or untreated until a later age. Clearly, health care providers, health care institutions, community-based organizations, and other social service agencies can play a very important role by educating parents that their children in the middle childhood, preadolescent, and adolescent years require access to health care and preventive services. Health care delivery systems also need to consider revising their standards of care and recommendations about needed health care services during the middle childhood and preadolescent years.

Middle childhood is also a good time to address or prevent obesity and eating disorders, such as anorexia and bulimia. Most obese adolescents do not become obese adults, but about 15 percent (well over the chance level) do become obese (Garn, 1992). This statistic merits attention in view of the long-term risks associated with obesity in adolescence, including cardiovascular disease and Type II diabetes. Parents, health professionals, and teachers can introduce or reinforce the importance of regular exercise and a good diet. Neither is sufficient alone for staying healthy throughout the life span; they must be considered together. Again, health care providers, social agencies, educators, and community-based programs can and should be playing an active role to ensure that adolescents know what constitutes a healthful diet and are encouraged to eat well-balanced meals and exercise regularly. They are also often in a unique position to identify children and adolescents who are at high risk for developing an eating disorder before they develop such problems and to ensure that children and adolescents who do have an eating disorder know how to get help.

Storm and stress are not inevitable in adolescence. The developmental milestones of adolescence have often been viewed in terms of pathology, yet decades of research would suggest otherwise. It is important to communicate clearly that adolescence does not inevitably bring on years of storm and stress for young people or their families. A classic epidemiological study of the mental health status of adolescents conducted in Great Britain by Michael Rutter and his colleagues found that half reported sadness or "misery" on questionnaires, but less than 15 percent of boys or girls were found to be depressed—that is, to have impaired functioning or true mood disturbance—based on in-depth interviews (Rutter et al., 1976).

When psychological difficulties do occur in adolescence, they are not necessarily outgrown later. At the same time, there has been a growing recognition from the past decade of research that psychological difficulties during adolescence need and deserve attention from parents and professionals. When adults overlook these problems, assuming that they are an inevitable part of adolescence and will be outgrown, they may be placing young people at risk; there is evidence that difficulties experienced in adolescence often continue into adulthood (Petersen, 1988). Will and commitment on the part of society are needed to screen for and respond to mental health problems experienced by adolescents to ensure that they do not become chronic and debilitating problems in adulthood.

Biology is not destiny. Although it gives definition to various aspects of development, biology alone does not determine outcomes (positive or negative) for young people. The modern perspective is that behavioral factors also modulate biological systems. It is widely recognized that many factors—including some that parents can influence—affect the course of adolescent development. Genetic differences among individuals and groups are usually influenced by social and cultural contexts. For example, differences in the timing of puberty for black and white girls may relate only partially to genetic factors; nutrition, socioeconomic conditions, and other factors have been shown to influence pubertal development.

Families matter. Humans are a social species. The regulation of children's biological systems, and their resilience when confronted with day-to-day stress, depend heavily on their interactions with important adults. This is true for adolescents as well as for younger children. Parents need to stay actively involved as their children move through the second decade. And although adolescents need and deserve privacy in some areas of their lives, stable, supportive relationships with parents and other family members are essential to their development, health, and well-being.

Civic engagement should be encouraged among adolescents. During the past two decades, there has been a growing literature that suggests that as much as 40 percent of young adolescents' time is unstructured, unsupervised, and consequently unproductive; much of this time occurs during the after-school hours when adolescents are frequently alone, watching television. Quite often, there are few after-school activities that provide young people with the opportunity to explore the community, put lessons learned in school and home to practical use, meet peers and adults other than classmates and teachers, and begin to transition to young adulthood (Carnegie Corporation of New York, 1995). Moreover, there are few links between schools and the workforce. Research shows that many factors influence adolescent development. Social institutions, such as schools, the health care delivery system, faith institutions, and community organizations, play an important role in supporting the healthy and productive development of adolescents. In this regard, adults appear to be missing important opportunities to influence young people's lives. In particular, research suggests, community context influences the developmental processes that can promote positive developmental outcomes among adolescents and discourage them from engaging in problem behaviors, such as substance abuse, precocious sexual activity, and delinquency (National Research Council, 1993, 1996; Petersen et al., 1991).

CONCLUSION

Other than infancy, no stage in human development results in such rapid or dramatic change than adolescence. During adolescence, a child matures into an adult physically. Within a matter of four to five years, the average child grows nearly a foot taller, assuming adult size, shape, and reproductive status. How can such enormous changes take place during such a compressed period? How does the body initiate, regulate, and time these changes? How do these changes affect behavior, and vice versa? Today, we are in a better position to answer these questions than ever before. Breakthroughs in science and technology have sparked an explosion of new knowledge about the developmental changes that occur during adolescence. Advances in neuroendocrinology and brain imaging are beginning to produce important insights into pubertal growth and adolescent development.

While focusing on the biological mechanisms that underlie adolescent development, workshop participants repeatedly sounded this theme: social ecology is crucial. Physical development is influenced by a broad spectrum of environmental, social, and cultural factors, and both experience and heredity affect the timing of puberty. The evidence for this dual influence is growing rapidly.

The study of adolescence in general, and puberty in particular, is challenging as a result of their complexity. A multitude of factors interact, affecting the timing and trajectory of development in the second decade of life. Which factors interact under which circumstances? Which factors are driving forces in adolescent development, and which have more marginal roles? What is the relationship between the timing of puberty and the progression of hormonal changes? These are some of the issues that will require further investigation as the field of adolescent development itself comes of age.

REFERENCES

Brooks-Gunn, J., J.A. Graber, and R.L. Paikoff
  1994 Studying links between hormones and negative affect: Models and measures. *Journal of Research on Adolescence* 4(4):469-486.
Brooks-Gunn, J., and E.O. Reiter
  1990 The role of pubertal processes in early adolescent transition. In *At the Threshold: The Developing Adolescent*, S. Feldman and G. Elliott, eds. Cambridge: Harvard University Press.
Brown, K.M., R.P. McMahon, F.M. Biro, P. Crawford, G.B. Schreiber, S.L. Similo, M. Waclawiw, and R. Striegel-Moore
  1998 Changes in self-esteem in black and white girls between the ages of 9 and 14 years: The NHLBI Growth and Health Study. *Journal of Adolescent Health*, February 22(2):7-19.
Buchanan, C.M., J.S. Eccles, and J.B. Becker
  1992 Are adolescents the victims of raging hormones? Evidence of activational effects of hormones on moods and behavior at adolescence. *Psychological Bulletin* 111(1):62-107.
Carnegie Corporation of New York
  1995 *Great Transitions: Preparing Adolescents for a New Century.* Carnegie Council on Adolescent Development. New York: Carnegie Corporation of New York.
Caspi, A., D. Lynam, T.E. Moffitt, and P.A. Silva
  1993 Unraveling girls' delinquency: Biological, dispositional, and contextual contributions to adolescent misbehavior. *Developmental Psychology* 29(1):19-30.
Crockett, L.J., and A.C. Petersen
  1993 Adolescent development: Health risks and opportunities for health promotion. In *Promoting the Health of Adolescents*, S.G. Millstein, A.C. Petersen, and E.O. Nightingale, eds. New York, NY: Oxford University Press
Dorn, L.D., L.J. Crockett, and A.C. Petersen
  1988 The relations of pubertal status to intrapersonal changes in young adolescents. *Journal of Early Adolescence* 8:405-419.
Elkind, D.
  1992 Cognitive development. In *Comprehensive Adolescent Health Care*, S.B. Friedman, M. Fisher, and S. Kenneth Schonberg, eds. St. Louis, MO: Quality Medical Publishing, Inc.
Flannery, D.J., D.C. Rowe, and B.L. Gulley
  1993 Impact of pubertal status, timing, and age: Adolescent sexual experience and delinquency. *Journal of Adolescent Research* 8(1):21-40.
Garn, S.M.
  1992 Physical growth and development. In *Comprehensive Adolescent Health Care,* S.B. Friedman, M. Fisher, and S. Kenneth Schonberg, eds. St. Louis, MO: Quality Medical Publishing, Inc.
Ge, X., R.D. Conger, and G.H. Elder, Jr.
  1995 Coming of age too early: Pubertal influences on girls' vulnerability to psychological distress. *Child Development* 67:3386-3400.

Graber, J.A., and J. Brook-Gunn
    1999 Reproductive transitions: The experience of mothers and daughters. In *The Parental Experience in Midlife*, C.D. Ryff and M.M. Seltzer, eds. Chicago, IL: University of Chicago Press.

Graber, J.A., J. Brooks-Gunn, and M.P. Warren
    1995 The antecedents of menarcheal age: Heredity, family environment, and stressful life events. *Child Development* 66:346-359.

Graber, J.A., P.M. Lewinsohn, J.R. Seeley, and J. Brooks-Gunn
    1997 Is psychopathology associated with the timing of pubertal development? *Journal of the American Academy of Child and Adolescent Psychiatry* 36(12):1768-1776.

Graber, J.A., and Warren, M.P.
    1992 The Role of Adrenal Androgens in Psychosocial and Biological Development at Puberty. Paper presented at the biennial meeting of the Society for Research in Child Development, March, 1993. New Orleans, LA.

Grumbach, M.M., and D.M. Styne
    1998 Puberty and its disorders. In Williams' *Textbook of Endocrinology*, 9th ed. J.D. Wilson, D.W. Foster, H. Kronenberg, and P.R. Larsen, eds. Philadelphia: W.B. Saunders.

Hall, G.S.
    1904 *Adolescence: Its Psychology and Its Relations to Physiology, Anthropology, Sociology, Sex, Crime, Religion, and Education*, Vols. 1-2. New York: Appleton-Century-Crofts.

Hamburg, B.A.
    1992 Psychosocial development. In *Comprehensive Adolescent Health Care*, S.B. Friedman, M. Fisher, and S. Kenneth Schonberg, eds. St. Louis, MO: Quality Medical Publishing, Inc.

Hardy, J.B., S. Shapiro, N.M. Astone, T.L. Miller, J. Brooks-Gunn, and S.C. Hilton
    1997 Adolescent childbearing revisited: The age of inner-city mothers at delivery is a determinant of their children's self-sufficiency at age 27 to 33. *Pediatrics* 100(5):802-809.

Henshaw, S.K.
    1998 U.S. teenage pregnancy statistics. New York: Alan Guttmacher Institute.

Institute of Medicine
    1995 *The Best Intentions: Unintended Pregnancy and the Well-Being of Children and Families.* Committee on Unintended Pregnancy, Institute of Medicine. Washington, D.C.: National Academy Press.

Keenan, K., and D. Shaw
    1997 Developmental and social influences on young girls' early problem behavior. *Psychological Bulletin* 121(1):95-113.

Litt, I.F.
    1995 Pubertal and psychosocial development: Implications for pediatricians. *Pediatrics in Review* 16(7):243-247.

National Research Council
    1993 *Losing Generations: Adolescents in High-Risk Settings.* Panel on High Risk Youth, National Research Council. Washington, D.C.: National Academy Press.

1996 *Youth Development and Neighborhood Influences: Challenges and Opportunities.* Committee on Youth Development, National Research Council. Washington, D.C.: National Academy Press.

Petersen, A.C.
 1988 Adolescent development. *American Review of Psychology* 39:583-607.

Petersen, A.C., C.R. Bingham, M. Stemmler, and L.J. Crockett
 1991 Subcultural Variation in Developmental Processes: The Development of Depressed Affect. Paper presented at the 11th Biennial Meeting of the International Society for the Study of Behavioral Development, July 3-7, Minneapolis, Minnesota.

Petersen, A.C., and N. Leffert
 in press What is Special About Adolescence? Youth in the Year 2000: Psychosocial Issues and Interventions. Invited presentation at a conference sponsored by the Johann Jacobs Foundation at Marbach Castle, Germany, November, 1992. To be published in an untitled volume, M. Rutter, ed. London: Cambridge University Press.

Pusey, A.E.
 1990 Behavioural changes at adolescence in chimpanzees. *Behaviour* 115(3-4):203-246.

Raine, A., P.H. Venables, and M. Williams
 1997 High autonomic arousal and electrodermal orienting at age 15 years as protective factors against criminal behavior at age 29 years. *American Journal of Psychiatry* 152:11.

Richards, M.H., and R. Larson
 1993 Pubertal development and the daily subjective states of young adolescents. *Journal of Research on Adolescence* 3(2):145-169.

Rutter, M., H. Giller, and A. Hagell
 1998 *Antisocial Behavior by Young People.* New York: Cambridge University Press.

Rutter, M., P. Graham, and O.F.D. Chadwick
 1976 Adolescent turmoil: Fact or fiction. *Journal of Child Psychological Psychiatry* 17:35.

Rutter, M., and Smith, D., eds.
 1995 *Psychosocial Disorders of Young People: Time Trends and Their Causes.* New York: Wiley.

Suomi, S.J.
 1991 Adolescent depression and depressive symptoms: Insights from longitudinal studies with rhesus monkeys. *Journal of Youth and Adolescence* 20(2):273-286.
 1997 Early determinants of behaviour: Evidence from primate studies. *British Medical Bulletin* 53(1):170-184.

Susman, E.J.
 1997 Modeling developmental complexity in adolescence: Hormones and behavior in context. *Journal of Research on Adolescence* 7(3):286-306.

Susman, E.J., E.D Nottleman, L.D. Dorn, P.W. Gold, and G.P. Chrousos
 1989 The physiology of stress and behavioral development. In *Coping with Uncertainty: Behavioral and Developmental Perspectives,* D.S. Palermo, ed. Hillsdale, NJ: Lawrence Erlbaum Associates, Inc.

APPENDIX
WORKSHOP AGENDA

New Research on the Biology of Puberty and Adolescent Development

March 23 - 24, 1998

National Academy of Sciences/National Research Council
Washington, DC 20418

Monday, March 23
2101 Constitution Avenue, NAS Members Room
Chair: David Hamburg

6:00 - 7:30 p.m.	Reception and Dinner	
7:30 - 8:00 p.m.	Orientation to the Meeting	David Hamburg
8:00 - 8:45 p.m.	Overview: The Developing Adolescent	Anne Petersen

Tuesday, March 24
2001 Wisconsin Avenue - Green Building, Room 130
Chair: Melvin Grumbach

8:00 - 8:15 a.m.	Continental breakfast available	
8:15 - 8:50 a.m.	Pubertal Maturation Among Girls in the US	Frank Biro

Session I: Adolescence in Animals

8:50 - 9:15 a.m.	Behavioral and Physiological Changes Associated with Puberty in Non-human Primates	Steven Suomi
9:15 - 9:25 a.m.	Discussant	
9:25 - 9:55 a.m.	Open Discussion	Anne Pusey

Session II: Neuroendocrine Physiology at Puberty

9:55 - 10:20 a.m.	Paradigms and Progress in Hormone-behavior Interactions at Puberty	Elizabeth Susman
10:20 - 10:30 a.m.	Discussant	Iris Litt
10:30 - 11:00 a.m.	Open Discussion	

Session III: The Interplay Between Pubertal Development and Behavior

11:00 - 11:25 a.m.	Sexual Behavior	Jeanne Brooks-Gunn
11:25 - 11:50 a.m.	Aggressive/Problem Behavior	David Rowe
11:50 - 12:00 p.m.	Discussant	Ruth Gross
12:00 - 12:35 p.m.	Open Discussion	

Session IV: Implications for Research, Policy and Practice

12:35 - 1:30 p.m.	Working Lunch	
12:50 - 1:00 p.m.	Discussant	Huda Akil
1:00 - 2:00 p.m.	Open Discussion	
02:00 p.m.	Adjourn